MW00974949

Vegan

100% Gluten Free

Insanely Good and Healthy, Vegan Gluten Free Recipes for Weight Loss & Wellbeing

By <u>Karen Greenvang</u> (aka Karen Vegan)

Copyright ©Karen Greenvang 2016

www.HolisticWellnessBooks.com

All information in this book has been carefully researched and checked for factual accuracy. However, the author and publishers make no warranty, expressed or implied, that the information contained herein is appropriate for every individual, situation or purpose, and assume no responsibility for errors or omission. The reader assumes the risk and full responsibility for all actions, and the author will not be held liable for any loss or damage, whether consequential, incidental, and special or otherwise, that may result from the information presented in this publication.

All cooking is an experiment in a sense, and many people come to the same or similar recipe over time. All recipes in this book have been derived from author's personal experience. Should any bear a close resemblance to those used elsewhere, that is purely coincidental.

The book is not intended to provide medical advice or to take the place of medical advice and treatment from your personal physician. Readers are advised to consult their own doctors or other qualified health professionals regarding the treatment of medical conditions. The author shall not be held liable or responsible for any misunderstanding or misuse of the information contained in this book. The information is not intended to diagnose, treat or cure any disease.

It is important to remember that the author of this book is not a doctor/ medical professional. Only opinions based upon her own personal experiences or research are cited. THE AUTHOR DOES NOT OFFER MEDICAL ADVICE or prescribe any treatments. For any health or medical issues – you should be talking to your doctor first.

Table of Contents

Introduction: Vegan Gluten-Free Cooking

Gluten is a protein found in grains such as wheat, barley, rye and sometimes even oats. For those suffering from a gluten allergy, intolerance and the more serious coeliac disease, a diet that provides optimum nutrition and all your dietary needs has been very difficult to achieve in the past. This is because many commercially made foods contain fillers that are gluten based. Even the most common of condiments may contain maize starch, and anything that lists malt in its ingredients will be a gluten containing food.

Luckily the effects of gluten allergies, intolerances and coeliac disease have become better known to both consumers and manufacturers over the last few years, making gluten free options more available and more affordable than they previously were.

Whether one's choice to take on a lifestyle and diet that excludes all animal proteins and the plant protein gluten is as a means to treat and further prevent an existing diagnosed medical condition, or if it is just a choice you have made due to ethical and personal reasons, it is still imperative to make sure that you are feeding your body with the a nutritionally balanced and sound diet. One of the best ways to achieve this is by taking on the vegan clean eating approach and the best way to achieve this is by cooking and preparing all your foods yourself, sticking to basics and creating flavorful meals without any unnecessary harmful additives.

The recipes in this book are all vegan friendly and gluten-free, they are easy to prepare and use only natural and basic ingredients, with no unnecessary additives that are usually found in prepared commercial foods. The focus is on healthy, clean eating that provides sound nutrition without sacrificing flavor and comfort. 100% cruelty-free.

Now you can begin preparing healthy, tasty and nutritious meals without any concern that you may be ingesting foods that don't fit into your chosen lifestyle. This book is divided into four sections, Breakfasts, Lunches, Dinners and Snacks and therefore provides you with many options.

Enjoy!

Free Complimentary eBook

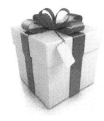

Before we dive into the recipes, I would like to offer you a free, complimentary recipe eBook with delicious vegan superfood smoothies.

Download it now, before you forget:

Download link: www.bitly.com/karenfreegift

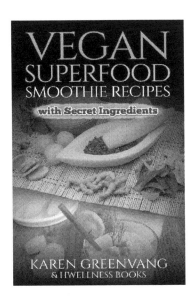

If you have any problems with your download, email me at:
karenveganbooks@gmail.com

Breakfasts

Breakfast is really the most important meal of the day. By starting every day off with a wholesome and nutritious breakfast that ideally contains a good balance of protein and carbohydrate, you are not only kick-starting your metabolism for the day, which is necessary in maintaining a healthy weight, but you are also giving your body the fuel it needs to help maintain healthy blood glucose levels. The recipes in this section are all easy to prepare, and some may even be prepared in advance for those quick run-out-the-door mornings. The combination of healthy proteins, carbohydrates and fats in every option will help you make sure that you get your day off to a healthy, nutritious start and avoid that mid-morning slump.

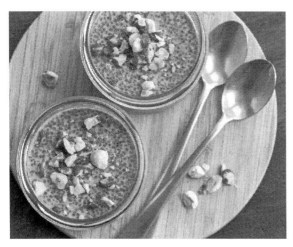

Breakfast Jars

The concept of a pre-made breakfast in a jar is incredibly versatile and time-saving, as it is something that you can prepare the night before and refrigerate until morning. Because the breakfast jar recipes that follow are made in a mason jar and are a gluten-free alternative based on the overnight oats concept, they are a perfect on-the-run breakfast option. The use of Chia seeds instead of oats provides a healthy dose of omega-3's and the added fruits bring in healthy carbohydrates, vitamins and minerals. Each jar is a single serving, so you would need to make one jar per person.

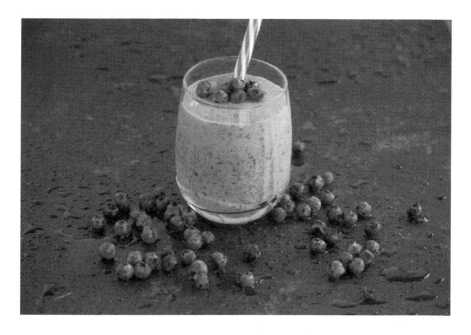

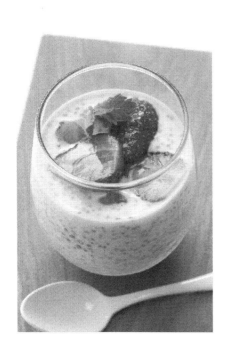

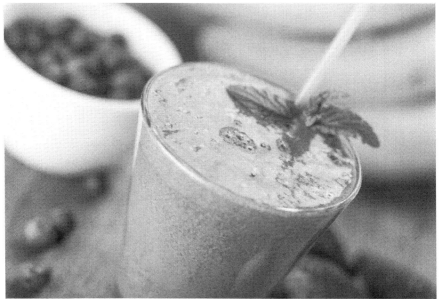

Carrot "Cake" Chia Seed Breakfast Jar

Carrots are a great source of vitamin A, are high in fiber, and a small amount of healthy carbohydrate. The golden sultanas not only add a hint of sweetness, but also are high in vitamin C. The coconut milk and pecan nuts provide a further dose of healthy fats and the ground ginger and cinnamon have anti-inflammatory and immune-boosting properties.

Serves One

Ingredients:

- 2 Tablespoons (30ml) Chia Seeds

- ¼ Cup (60ml) Coconut Milk

- 1 Tablespoon (15ml) Golden Sultanas

- 2 Teaspoons (10ml) Grated Carrot

- 1 Tablespoon (15ml) Raw pecan nuts, chopped

- ¼ Teaspoon (1.25ml) Ground Cinnamon

- ¼ Teaspoon (1.25ml) Baking spice mix

- ¼ Teaspoon (1.25ml) Ground Ginger

- ¼ Teaspoon (1.25ml) Vanilla Essence

Instructions:

1. In a medium-sized Mason jar, mix the Chia seeds, grated carrot, sultanas, ground cinnamon, baking spice mix, ground ginger, and pecan nuts.

2. In a small milk jug, mix the coconut milk with the vanilla essence and pour over the other ingredients that are already in the Mason jar.

3. Mix all ingredients well, making sure that everything is combined and place the lid tightly on the jar.

4. Refrigerate overnight.

5. The idea is to eat this breakfast out of the jar, and it can be served with ¼ cup (60ml) vegan yoghurt (like for example coconut yoghurt).

and Banana Chia Seed Breakfast Jar

a wonderful source of healthy carbohydrate and their high potassium content makes them an incredibly good source of pre and post workout energy. The almonds are high in healthy fats and protein. The raisins add a little extra sweetness and are a good source of energy and iron.

Serves One

Ingredients:

- 2 Tablespoons (30ml) Chia Seeds

- ¼ Cup (60ml) Almond Milk

- 1 Tablespoon (15ml) Raisins

- 1 small Banana, mashed

- 1 Tablespoon (15ml) Raw almonds, chopped (you can also use raw almond flakes)

- ¼ Teaspoon (1.25ml) Ground Cinnamon

- ¼ Teaspoon (1.25ml) Vanilla Essence

Instructions:

1. In a medium-sized Mason jar, mix the Chia seeds, raisins, mashed banana, ground cinnamon and almonds.

2. In a small milk jug, mix the almond milk with the vanilla essence and pour over the other ingredients that are already in the Mason jar.

3. Mix all ingredients well, making sure that everything is combined and place the lid tightly on the jar.

4. Refrigerate overnight.

5. The idea is to eat this breakfast out of the jar, and it can be served with ¼ cup (60ml) vegan yoghurt of your choice.

Apple Cinnamon Chia Seed Breakfast Jar

Apples are a great source of vitamin C, and their high pectin content makes them incredibly filling and satisfying, making this a fruit a great breakfast addition since it will keep you going all morning. The almond milk in this variation provides a healthy dose of calcium and protein, and by serving it with natural peanut butter you are getting a little extra protein and healthy fats.

Serves One

Ingredients:

- 2 Tablespoons (30ml) Chia Seeds

- ¼ Cup (60ml) Almond Milk

- 1 Tablespoon (15ml) Raisins

- 1 Tablespoon (15ml) Grated Apple

- ¼ Teaspoon (1.25ml) Ground Cinnamon

- ¼ Teaspoon (1.25ml) Baking Spice mix

- ¼ Teaspoon (1.25ml) Vanilla Essence

- 1 Teaspoon (5ml) Natural peanut butter (for serving)

Instructions:

1. In a medium-sized Mason jar, mix the Chia seeds, raisins, grated apple, ground cinnamon and baking spice mix.

2. In a small milk jug, mix the almond milk with the vanilla essence and pour over the other ingredients that are already in the Mason jar.

3. Mix all ingredients well, making sure that everything is combined and place the lid tightly on the jar.

4. Refrigerate overnight.

5. Top with the natural peanut butter before serving

6. The idea is to eat this breakfast out of the jar, and it can be served with ¼ cup (60ml) dairy-free vegan yoghurt of your choice.

Chocolate Berry Delight Chia Seed Breakfast Jar

Strawberries are rich in anti-oxidants and high in vitamin C. Raw cocoa is a super food that is also very high in antioxidants and known for its blood pressure reducing properties. Goji berries that are found in the dried berry mix are also considered a super food, and it is well known that Chia seeds carry the super food label, therefore this breakfast jar is a complete super food guaranteed to start your day in a super way.

Serves One

Ingredients:

- 2 Tablespoons (30ml) Chia Seeds

- ¼ Cup (60ml) Coconut Milk (can be also almond milk, chia seed milk, cashew milk etc.)

- 1 Tablespoon (15ml) Dried Berry mix

- 1 Tablespoon (15ml) Fresh Strawberries, finely chopped

- ¼ Teaspoon (1.25ml) Ground Cinnamon

- 1 Teaspoon (5ml) Raw Cocoa Powder

- ¼ Teaspoon (1.25ml) Vanilla Essence

Instructions:

1. In a medium-sized Mason jar, mix the Chia seeds, dried berry mix, chopped strawberries, ground cinnamon and raw cocoa powder.

2. In a small milk jug, mix the coconut milk with the vanilla essence and pour over the other ingredients that are already in the Mason jar.

3. Mix all ingredients well, making sure that everything is combined and place the lid tightly on the jar.

4. Refrigerate overnight.

5. The idea is to eat this breakfast out of the jar, and it can be served with ¼ cup (60ml) dairy-free vegan friendly yoghurt of your choice.

Cooked Breakfasts

The more relaxed weekend mornings lend themselves to the opportunity of spending some quality time in the kitchen preparing a healthy cooked breakfast option. Some of these recipes are served with gluten-free breads that are available in most health stores and many supermarkets nowadays, but of course the addition of such breads is entirely up to personal choice. The inclusion of tofu in some of these recipes provides a very healthy source of protein, as do those that include beans and legumes. The use of olive oil in some instances adds to the healthy fat content. Usually cooked breakfasts tend to be very heavy and are the reason why many people tend to skip breakfast, because they can't face a big meal first thing in the morning, but these recipes are light, and easy to prepare, providing breakfast options that will satisfy your hunger without weighing you down.

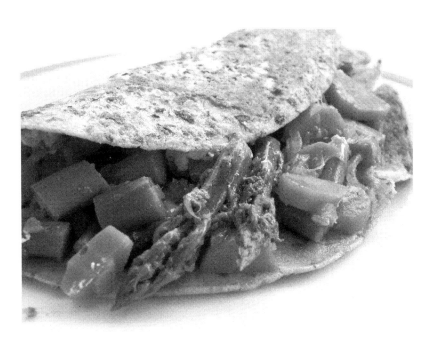

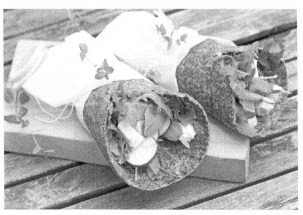

23

Tofu Scramble with Roasted Cherry Tomatoes

Tomatoes are very high in vitamin C as well as essential minerals. They are also high in the anti-oxidant lycopene, which is known for its bone-building properties. The cherry tomato variety adds a unique sweetness to the overall flavor of the dish. Research has shown that by cooking tomatoes in olive oil you increasing the body's ability to absorb the lycopene from the tomatoes. This is an incredibly nutritious, high protein breakfast option.

Serves One

Ingredients:

- ½ Cup (125ml) Firm Tofu, diced

- ½ Cup (125ml) Cherry tomatoes, halved

- ¼ Cup (60ml) Fresh avocado, diced

- 1 Tablespoon (15ml) Fresh Basil, chopped

- ½ Teaspoon (2.5ml) Ground Organic Sea Salt

- ½ Teaspoon (2.5ml) Ground Black Pepper

- 2 Tablespoons (30ml) Extra Virgin Organic Olive Oil

- 1 Slice gluten-free bread for serving (optional)

Instructions:

1. Preheat the oven to 350 degrees (200 degrees Celsius)

2. In a baking dish, combine the cherry tomatoes, ¼ teaspoon (1.25ml) of the ground sea salt, ¼ teaspoon (1,25ml) of the ground black pepper, the fresh basil and 1 tablespoon (15ml) of the olive oil. Roast in the oven until the tomatoes have softened completely, this should take at least 40 minutes.

3. In a mixing bowl, mix the diced tofu with the remaining tablespoon (15ml) of olive oil, ¼ teaspoon (1.25ml) ground sea salt, ¼ teaspoon (1.25ml) ground black pepper, and fry in a non-stick pan or wok until the tofu is golden brown.

4. Place the roasted cherry tomatoes on a plate and top with the cooked tofu and diced avocado. Serve hot.

5. If you choose to include the gluten-free bread, then that will be placed on the plate first, then topped with the cherry tomatoes, tofu and avocado.

6. It is also optional to drizzle a little organic extra virgin olive oil over the top of this meal before serving.

Seared Tofu with Black Mushrooms and Mustard Micro Greens

Mushrooms are a great source of the minerals iron and selenium. The mustard micro greens add a unique flavor to this dish. Once again you can choose whether or not to serve this dish with a gluten-free bread option.

Serves One

Ingredients:

- Two thick slices of firm tofu

- 1 Cup (250ml) Fresh black mushrooms, chopped

- 1 Tablespoon (15ml) Fresh Garlic, finely chopped

- 1 Teaspoon (5ml) Dried Italian Herb mix

- ¼ Teaspoon (1.25ml) Ground Organic Sea Salt

- ¼ Teaspoon (1.25ml) Ground Black Pepper

- 1 Tablespoon (15ml) Mustard Micro Greens

Instructions:

1. In a saucepan, combine the chopped black mushrooms, garlic, salt, pepper and dried herb mix. Cook on a low

heat for about 30 minutes, until the mushrooms have completely reduced and almost formed their own stock.

2. In a non-stick pan, lightly sear the tofu slices until golden brown on all sides

3. Place the cooked black mushrooms on a plate and top with the seared tofu slices

4. Garnish with mustard micro greens

5. Serve with gluten-free bread of your choice (optional)

Lunches

What makes lunch such an important meal in the day is the fact that it's what breaks a busy day in half, allowing us time to re-energize and refuel our bodies in order to continue through the day at our best. Because lunchtime is our re-fueling pit stop, it important to make sure that we have a well-balanced, nutritious meal that includes sufficient protein and carbohydrate. The recipes in this section are light, and easy to prepare in advance, making them great lunch box options that will help you ensure that you are getting a midday meal that meets your unique dietary requirements.

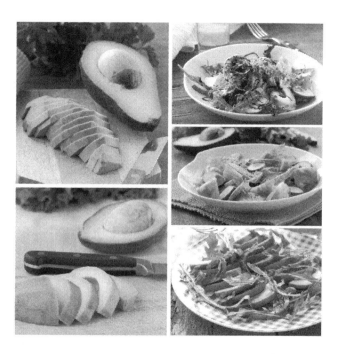

Quinoa, Kidney Bean and Baby Spinach Salad

Quinoa is a gluten free grain that is known for its high fiber and protein content, the red kidney beans not only add a dash of color to this salad, but they also bring in an extra source of protein, fiber and healthy carbohydrate. The raw baby spinach is loaded with iron and essential minerals. The seed mix adds some healthy fats, as does the olive oil.

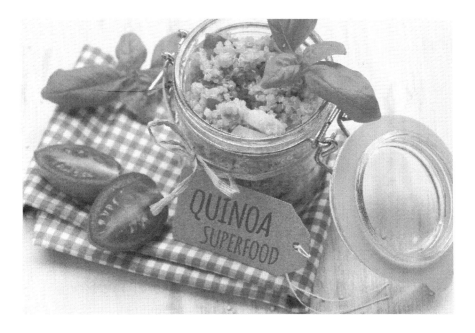

Serves One

Ingredients:

- ½ Cup (125ml) Cooked Quinoa

- ¼ Cup (60ml) Red Kidney beans (these can be the canned variety, make sure you rinse them well to wash away any excess sodium)

- 1 Cup (250ml) Raw Baby Spinach leaves

- 1 Tablespoon (15ml) Raw Seed Mix

- 1 Tablespoon (15ml) Organic Extra Virgin Olive Oil

- Ground black pepper and ground organic sea salt to taste

Instructions:

1. In a bowl, or a take-away tub if you are packing this lunch for work, place the cooked quinoa

2. Add the baby spinach leaves

3. Add the red kidney beans

4. Sprinkle the raw seed mix over the other ingredients, followed by the sea salt and black pepper

5. Just before serving, drizzle with the extra virgin olive oil and toss well

Roast Butternut, Beetroot and Chickpea Salad with Fresh Kale and Mustard Micro Greens

Butternut is high in vitamin A and beetroot is known for its high vitamin C content as well as its cancer fighting properties. The chickpeas add a wholesome source of protein and the mustard micro greens add to the flavor. This is another of those delicious salads that can be easily pre-packed for an office lunch.

Serves One

Ingredients:

- ½ Cup (125ml) Roasted Butternut

- ½ Cup (125ml) Roasted Beetroot

- ¼ Cup (60ml) Chickpeas (these can be the canned variety, just make sure they are well rinsed to ensure all excess sodium is washed away)

- ½ Cup (125ml) Fresh Raw Kale

- 1 Tablespoon (15ml) Raw Seed Mix

- 1 Tablespoon (15ml) Mustard Micro Greens

Instructions:

1. In a serving bowl, or a take-away tub, place the raw kale leaves

2. Add the roast butternut and beetroot

3. Add the chick peas

4. Sprinkle the raw seed mix and mustard micro greens over the top and toss well before serving.

Fresh Basil, Cherry Tomato and Herbed Tofu Salad with Pine nuts

There is just something amazing about the flavor combination of tomato and basil. This salad is a tasty, nutritious reason to take a break from your desk.

Serves One:

Ingredients:

- 1 Cup (250ml) Cooked, diced firm tofu

- ½ Cup (125ml) Fresh Basil leaves

- ½ Cup (125ml) Cherry tomatoes, halved

- 1 Tablespoon (15ml) Raw Pine nuts

- 2 Teaspoons (10ml) Organic Extra Virgin Olive Oil

Instructions:

1. In a serving bowl, or take away tub, place the fresh basil leaves

2. Add the halved cherry tomatoes

3. Add the cooked tofu

4. Top with the raw pine nuts

5. Just before serving drizzle with the olive oil and toss well. Salt and pepper can be added to taste.

Red Cabbage, Chick Pea and Pom
Salad with Pomegranate dres

Red cabbage not only provides great color to this c   _ it is
high in fiber, so will help keep you full all afternoon.
Pomegranates are high in antioxidants and are considered a
super food.

Serves One:

Ingredients for the salad:

- 1 Cup (250ml) Raw Red Cabbage, shredded

- ½ Cup (125ml) Chick peas (can be the canned variety, just make sure you rinse them well)

- ¼ Cup (60ml) Pomegranate Seeds

- 1 Tablespoon (15ml) Raw Seed Mix

Ingredients for the dressing:

- ¼ Cup (60ml) Fresh pomegranate juice

- 1 Tablespoon (15ml) Extra Virgin Coconut Oil

- ¼ Teaspoon (1.25ml) Organic Ground Sea Salt

- ¼ Teaspoon (1.25ml) Ground Black Pepper

ructions to make the salad:

1. In a serving bowl, or a take away tub, place the raw red cabbage

2. Add the chick peas

3. Add the pomegranate seeds

4. Add the raw seed mix

Instructions to make the dressing:

1. In a large mixing jug combine the pomegranate juice, coconut oil, salt and pepper.

2. Whisk well

3. Just before serving, pour the dressing over the salad and toss together

Buckwheat, Tofu, Pineapple and Cashew Nut Salad with a hint of Mint

Buckwheat is gluten-free grain that is high in fiber and is a great source of magnesium, it is also well known for its blood sugar regulating properties, making it a great lunch time choice in order to avoid the mid-afternoon slump. Pineapple is high in vitamin C and essential minerals, and the cashew nuts provide a nutritious crunch as well as a dose of healthy fats. The addition of fresh mint adds a light freshness to this salad, and also aids digestion.

Serves One

Ingredients for the salad:

- ½ Cup (125ml) Cooked Buckwheat

- ½ Cup (125ml) Cooked firm tofu, diced

- ¼ Cup (60ml) Fresh pineapple, diced

- 1 Tablespoon (15ml) Raw cashew nut halves

- 1 Tablespoon (15ml) Fresh mint leaves, chopped

Ingredients for the dressing:

- ¼ Cup (60ml) Fresh pineapple juice

- 1 Tablespoon (15ml) Extra Virgin Coconut Oil

- 1 Tablespoon (15ml) Desiccated Coconut

Instructions to make the salad:

1. In a serving bowl or take away tub, place the cooked buckwheat

2. Add the cooked, diced tofu

3. Add the fresh pineapple, and sprinkle the cashew nuts and chopped mint over the top

Instructions to make the dressing:

1. In a large mixing jug combine the pineapple juice, coconut oil and desiccated coconut

2. Whisk well

3. Just before serving the salad, pour the dressing over the top and toss together

Cucumber, Kale and Lentil Salad

Cucumbers are known for their ability to combat dehydration, making them a great lunchtime addition to combat all those morning cups of coffee. Lentils are a great source of protein and fiber and the kale is rich in essential minerals. The pumpkin seeds are high in omega fats and essential minerals.

Serves One

Ingredients:

- ½ Cup (125ml) Raw Kale

- ½ Cup (125ml) Lentils, (these can be the canned variety, just make sure that they have been well rinsed)

- ¼ Cup (60ml) Fresh cucumber, thinly sliced

- 1 Tablespoon (15ml) Raw Pumpkin Seeds

Instructions:

1. In a serving bowl, or take away tub, place the raw kale leaves

2. Add the lentils and cucumber slices

3. Sprinkle the pumpkin seeds over the top and toss together.

Teff, Tofu and Coriander Salad with Mung Bean Sprouts and Raw Peanuts

Teff is another gluten-free grain that is very high in calcium and is also an excellent source of vitamin C, which is not usually a vitamin found in grains. Coriander is a great source of essential minerals and vitamin K. The raw peanuts add a healthy crunch and a nutty flavor to the whole meal and the golden sultanas bring a hint of sweetness.

Serves One

Ingredients:

- ½ Cup (125ml) Cooked Teff (can be replaced with quinoa or amaranth)

- ½ Cup (125ml) Cooked firm tofu, diced

- ¼ Cup (60ml) Mung Bean Sprouts

- ¼ Cup (60ml) Fresh Coriander

- 1Tablespoon (15ml) Raw peanuts, chopped

- 1 Tablespoon (15ml) Golden Sultanas

Instructions:

1. In a serving bowl or take away tub, place the cooked Teff

2. Add the cooked tofu

3. Add the Mung bean sprouts and fresh coriander

4. Sprinkle over the raw peanuts and sultanas

5. Toss together and serve

e, Roast Egg Plant and Zucchini
th Black Olives and Chickpeas

other of the gluten-free grains that is high in vitamin B and essential minerals. Egg plants are a great source of dietary fiber and phytonutrients. Zucchini are a great source of manganese and the black olives not only add unique flavor but are also packed with heart healthy fats.

Serves One

Ingredients:

- ½ Cup (125ml) Cooked Brown Rice

- ½ Cup (135ml) Roasted Egg Plant

- ½ Cup (125ml) Roasted Zucchini

- ¼ Cup (60ml) Chickpeas (these can be the canned variety, just make sure that they have been well rinsed)

- ¼ Cup (60ml) Pitted Black Olives

- 1 Tablespoon (15ml) Extra Virgin Olive oil

- ¼ Teaspoon (1,25ml) Ground organic sea salt

- ¼ Teaspoon (1.25ml) Ground Black Pepper

Instructions to roast the eggplant and Zucchini:

1. Preheat the oven to 350 degrees (200degrees Celsius)

2. Dice the eggplant and thinly slice the zucchini

3. Place the eggplant and zucchini in and oven proof dish and toss with the extra virgin olive oil, sea salt and black pepper

4. Roast in the oven for about 40 minutes, allow to cool

Instructions to make the salad:

1. In a serving bowl or a take away tub, place the cooked brown rice

2. Add the roasted eggplant and zucchini

3. Add the chickpeas

4. Top with the black olives, toss together and serve

Red Cabbage, Apple and Walnut Salad with Chickpeas and Mustard Micro Greens

This is a crunchy salad that combines the spiciness of the raw cabbage and the sweetness of the apples. The walnuts add a nutty crunch as well as their nutritional benefits of omega 3 fats and their cholesterol controlling properties. The mustardy hint that is given by the micro greens rounds the flavors off nicely and the raisins add a little chewy sweetness.

Serves One

Ingredients:

- 1 Cup (250ml) Raw Red Cabbage, shredded

- 1 medium sized Green Apple, thinly sliced

- 1 Tablespoon (15ml) freshly squeezed lemon juice

- ¼ Cup (60ml) Chickpeas (these can be the canned variety, just make sure they are well rinsed)

- 1 Tablespoon (15ml) Raw Walnuts, roughly chopped

- 1 Tablespoon (15ml) Mustard Micro Greens

- 1 Tablespoon (15ml) Raisins

Instructions:

1. In a serving bowl or take away tub, place the red cabbage

2. Add the sliced apple and pour the lemon juice over it to ensure that the apple doesn't brown

3. Add the chickpeas

4. Add the roughly chopped walnuts

5. Add the Mustard Micro Greens

6. Add the raisins

7. Toss together and serve.

Lentil, Carrot and Pineapple Salad with Brazil Nuts

The combination of carrot and pineapple in this salad has a refreshing taste that will be sure to re-energize you and give you the kick you need to take on the rest of the afternoon. Brazil nuts are known for their high selenium contents, making them a very healthy fat addition. They also add a nutty crunch.

Serves One

Ingredients:

- ½ Cup (125ml) Cooked Quinoa

- ½ Cup (125ml) Lentils, (these can be the canned variety, just make sure that they are well rinsed)

- ½ Cup (125ml) Fresh Carrot, grated

- ¼ Cup (60ml) Fresh Pineapple, chopped

- 1 Tablespoon (15ml) Raw Brazil nuts, chopped

- 1 Tablespoon (15ml) Golden Sultanas

Instructions:

1. In a serving bowl or take away tub, place the cooked quinoa

2. Add the lentils

3. Add the grated carrot

4. Add the fresh pineapple and sprinkle over the chopped Brazil nuts and sultanas

5. Toss together and serve

Dinners

In our fast paced modern lifestyles, dinner is usually the only meal of the day that many families are actually able to share. Dinner time is also a time to unwind and refuel your body before retiring for the night. What makes dinner just as important a meal as the other two set meals in the day, is that it provides your body with sustenance to get you through the fast of sleeping, keeping your metabolism firing throughout the night and preventing blood sugar dips while you are sleeping. As with all the recipes in this book, these dishes are easy to prepare and will provide you and your family with a balanced, healthy meal at the end of each day.

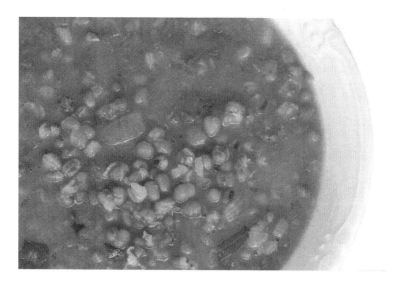

Curried Butternut with Chickpeas, Brown Rice and Coconut Milk

This is a comforting, well rounded meal that is perfect for winter nights. It does take some pre-preparation of the butternut and the brown rice, but once you have that cooked and available putting the rest of the dish together is quick and easy. The combination of healthy, slow releasing carbohydrates, protein and fats in this dish will keep you full throughout the night, avoiding that midnight hunger pang.

Serves 4

Ingredients:

- 2 Cups (500ml) Cooked Brown rice

- 2 Cups (500ml) Canned Chickpeas, drained and rinsed (you will probably need to cans to make up the 2 Cups)

- 4 Cups (1litre) Butternut, diced

- 1 Tablespoon (15ml) Extra Virgin Coconut Oil

- 1 Teaspoon (5ml) Gluten-free Masala Mix

- ½ Teaspoon (2.5ml) Ground Cinnamon

- ¼ Teaspoon (1.25ml) Cumin Seeds

- ¼ Teaspoon (1.25ml) Ground Coriander

- 2 Cups (500ml) Coconut Milk

- 4 Tablespoons (60ml) Desiccated Coconut

Instructions to cook the butternut:

1. Preheat the oven to 350 degrees (200 degrees Celsius)

2. Grease and oven proof dish with the coconut oil

3. Place the butternut into the dish and sprinkle with the Masala mix, ground cinnamon, cumin seeds and ground coriander.

4. Mix all together making sure that all the butternut is well covered with the spices

5. Roast for about 1 hour until the butternut has softened and browned

Instructions to make the full dish:

1. Preheat the oven to 350 degrees (200 degrees Celsius)

2. Using four separate single serving oven proof dishes, place ½ cup (125ml) of the cooked brown rice in each dish

3. Add ½ cup (125ml) Chickpeas to each dish

4. Add 1 cup (250ml) of the roasted butternut to each dish

5. Pour ½ cup (125ml) of the coconut milk over each dish

6. Sprinkle 1 tablespoon (15ml) of the desiccated coconut over each dish

7. Cover the dishes and bake in the oven for 40 minutes.

8. Since each serving is in its own dish already, this meal can be served straight from the oven.

Quinoa with Oven Roasted Sweet Peppers, Spinach, Tomatoes and Red Kidney Beans

This is another dish that requires some pre-preparation of the oven roasted vegetables and quinoa. The roasted sweet peppers and tomatoes provide a boost of vitamin C, while the spinach provides essential minerals such as iron. This dish is another wholesome dinner that is guaranteed to keep you and your family satisfied until breakfast time.

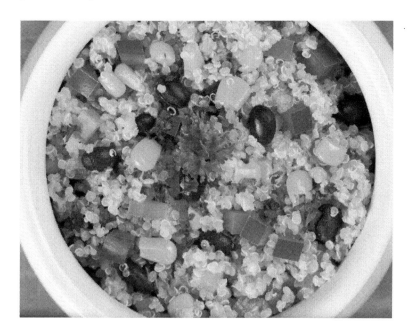

Serves 4

Ingredients:

- 4 Cups (1litre) Fresh Spinach, chopped

- 4 Cups (1litre) Mixed sweet peppers, chopped (make sure you have a variety of colors such as red, yellow, orange and green)

- 4 Cups (1litre) Cherry tomatoes, halved

- 1 Tablespoon (15ml) Fresh Garlic, finely chopped

- 1 Tablespoon (15ml) Fresh Basil leaves, finely chopped

- 1 teaspoon (5ml) Fresh Rosemary

- 1 teaspoon (5ml) Ground Black Pepper

- 1 teaspoon (5ml) Ground Organic Sea Salt

- 1 Tablespoon (15ml) Extra Virgin Olive Oil

- 2 Cups (500ml) Cooked quinoa

- 2 Cups (500ml) Canned Red Kidney beans, drained and rinsed (you may need two cans to make up the 2 Cups)

- 4 Tablespoons (60ml) Black olives, pitted

Instructions to make the oven roasted vegetables:

1. Preheat the oven to 350 degrees (200 degrees Celsius)

2. Grease a large roasting pan with the extra virgin olive oil

3. Place the chopped garlic, basil, rosemary, black pepper and sea salt in the bottom of the roasting pan

4. Place the chopped spinach into the roasting pan and then add the sweet peppers, followed by the cherry tomatoes

5. Toss all together and roast in the oven for 50 minutes

6. Once the 50 minutes has passed, switch off the oven and allow the vegetables to cool in the oven.

Instructions to make the full dish:

1. Preheat the oven to 350 degrees (200 degrees Celsius)

2. Using four separate single serving oven proof dishes, place ½ cup (125ml) of the cooked quinoa in each dish

3. Place 1 Cup (250ml) of the oven roasted vegetables in each dish

4. Place ½ Cup (125ml) of the red kidney beans in each dish

5. Top each dish with 1 tablespoon (15ml) of the pitted black olives

6. Bake in the oven for 20 minutes.

7. Since each serving is in its own dish already, this meal can be served straight from the oven.

Stuffed Egg Plant with Buckwheat, Cherry Tomatoes and Lentils

Egg Plant is a very filling and versatile vegetable, as this recipe shows. Once again, some pre-preparation is required here, but your efforts are guaranteed to produce a very wholesome and satisfying, balanced meal for your family.

Serves 4

Ingredients:

- 2 Large Egg plants

- 1 Cup (250ml) Cooked Buckwheat

- 1 Cup (250ml) Cherry tomatoes, halved

- 1 Cup (250ml) Canned Lentils, drained and rinsed

- 2 Tablespoons (30ml) Extra Virgin Olive oil

- 1 Tablespoon (15ml) Fresh Garlic, finely chopped

- 1 Tablespoon (15ml) Fresh Basil, finely chopped

- 1 Teaspoon (5ml) Fresh Rosemary

- 1 Teaspoon (5ml) Ground Black Pepper

- 1 Teaspoon (5ml) Ground Organic Sea Salt

- 4 Tablespoons (60ml) Black Olives, pitted and chopped

Instructions:

1. Preheat the oven to 350 degrees (200 degrees Celsius)

2. Cut the egg plants in half and scoop out the flesh, leaving just the shells.

3. Finely dice the eggplant flesh and place in a separate bowl

4. Using 1 Tablespoon (15ml) of the olive oil, grease an oven proof dish

5. Use the second tablespoon (15ml) of the olive oil to brush over the eggplant shells

6. Place the eggplant shells in the oven proof dish and cook for 25 minutes

7. To the separate bowl that contains the diced eggplant flesh, add the cooked quinoa, lentils, cherry tomatoes, salt, pepper, basil and rosemary. Mix together.

8. Once the eggplant shells come out of the oven begin to stuff them by scooping the mixture from step number 7 into each shell, making sure each is filled completely.

9. Top each stuffed eggplant shell with 1 tablespoon (15ml) of the black olive.

10. Drizzle a little extra virgin olive oil over each stuffed eggplant and place back in the oven for a further 30 minutes.

11. Serve with a green salad.

Cashew Nut Tofu with Brown Rice, Pineapple and Coconut Milk

This dish is inspired by the flavors commonly known to Thai dishes. It's a great way to add variety to the week's dinners and provides a very healthy balance of carbohydrates, protein, fats and the added bonus of fruit in the form of the pineapple. The hint of green chili gives it a little bite, without sacrificing flavor for fire.

Serves 4

Ingredients:

- 2 Cups (500ml) Cooked Brown Rice

- 4 Cups (1litre) Firm Tofu, diced

- 1 Cup (250ml) Fresh pineapple, cubed

- 2 Cups (500ml) Coconut Milk

- 4 Tablespoons (60ml) Raw Whole Cashew Nuts

- 1 Tablespoon (15ml) Freshly squeezed lime juice

- 1 teaspoon (5ml) Fresh green chili, finely chopped

- 1 Tablespoon (15ml) Fresh ginger root, finely chopped

- 1 Tablespoon (15ml) Fresh garlic, finely chopped

- 1 Tablespoon (15ml) Spring onions, finely chopped

- 1 Tablespoon (15ml) Extra Virgin Coconut Oil

Instructions:

1. Preheat the oven to 350 degrees (200degrees Celsius)

2. Heat the coconut oil in a wok and fry up the garlic, chili, ginger and spring onions

3. Add the tofu and lime juice

4. Continue to cook until the tofu has a golden brown finish

5. Using four separate single serving oven proof dishes, place ½ cup (125ml) of the cooked brown rice into each dish

6. Add 1 Cup (250ml) of the cooked tofu to each dish

7. Add ¼ cup (60ml) of the fresh pineapple to each dish

8. Add 1 tablespoon (15ml) of the raw cashew nuts to each dish

9. Pour ½ cup (125ml) of the coconut milk over each dish

10. Cover the dishes and bake in the oven for 30 minutes

11. Since each serving is in its own dish already, this meal can be served straight from the oven.

em Squash Stuffed with Lentils and Sweet Potato

Gem squash is high in carotene, which is known for its ability to aid the prevention of various heart diseases, they also contain a considerable amount of plant protein. Sweet potatoes provide a good dose of essential minerals and healthy, slow releasing carbohydrates. The combination of ingredients in this dish ensures another wholesome dinner that will comfort and satisfy your family's appetite to ensure a good night's rest. If gem squash is not easily available, this recipe can be made with any other similar type of small squash that is ideally the size of a softball, carnival squash would be another example.

Serves 4

Ingredients:

- 4 Medium sized Gem Squash

- 1 Cup (250ml) Canned lentils, drained and well rinsed

- 1 Large sweet potato

- 4 Tablespoons (60ml) Raw seed mix

- 1 Teaspoon (5ml) Extra Virgin olive oil

- 1 Teaspoon(5ml) Organic dried Italian herb mix

- ½ Teaspoon (2.5ml) Ground organic sea salt

- ½ Teaspoon (2.5ml) Ground black pepper

Instructions:

1. Preheat the oven to 350 degrees (200 degrees Celsius)

2. Cut each gem squash in half and scoop out the seeds

3. Place the gem squash halves in an oven proof dish and bake for 20 minutes

4. Dice the sweet potato (no need to peel it as this ensures that you don't lose the essential nutrients that are found just under the skin, but be sure to wash it well)

5. Place the sweet potato in a sauce pan with the organic sea salt and enough water to cover the potato, bring to the boil

6. Allow the sweet potato to simmer on a low heat until it has cooked to a very soft consistency

7. Once the sweet potato is cooked, drain off the water and return it to the saucepan

8. Add the dried Italian herb mix, black pepper and extra virgin olive oil

9. Mash the sweet potato mix until smooth

10. Once the gem squash halves come out of the oven begin to stuff them

11. Place ¼ cup (60ml) of the lentils into each gem squash half

12. Top each gem squash half with ¼ cup (60ml) of the mashed sweet potato

13. Sprinkle 1 tablespoon (15ml) of the raw seed mix over each of the gem squash halves

14. Drizzle a little extra olive oil over each gem squash half and bake in the oven for a further 40 minutes

15. Using four separate dinner plates place two gem squash halves on each plate and serve with a green salad.

Vegetable Pot Pie

This is an incredibly comforting meal that is great for winter nights. The high fiber and protein content ensures another satisfying dinner that is highly nutritious and also combines a variety of ingredients for great flavor.

Serves 4

Ingredients:

- 4 large sweet potatoes
- 2 Cups (500ml) Canned Red Kidney Beans
- 2 Cups (500ml) Diced butternut
- 2 Cups (500ml) Cherry tomatoes, halved
- 2 Cups (500ml) Cooked Quinoa
- 2 Teaspoons (10ml) Extra Virgin Olive Oil
- 1 Teaspoon (5ml) Dried Organic Italian Herb Mix
- 1 Teaspoon (5ml) Ground Organic Sea salt
- 1 Teaspoon (5ml) Ground Black Pepper
- 4 Tablespoons (60ml) Raw Seed mix

Instructions:

- Preheat the oven to 350 degrees (200 degrees Celsius)

- Dice the sweet potatoes (there is no need to peel them, as this ensures that you don't lose the essential minerals that are found just beneath the skin, just make sure that they are well washed)

- Place the sweet potatoes in a saucepan and cover with water, add the sea salt and bring to the boil

- Allow the sweet potatoes to simmer at a low heat until very soft

- Once the sweet potatoes are cooked, drain them and return them to the saucepan

- Add the ground black pepper, dried herb mix and olive oil

- Mash until smooth

- Place the diced butternut in a saucepan with water and bring to the boil

- Allow the butternut to simmer on a low heat until just soft enough (ideally a piece of butternut will remain on a fork for just a second before falling off, this is when it is ready)

- Drain the butternut and return it to the saucepan

- Using four separate single serving oven proof dishes, place ½ cup (250ml) of the cooked quinoa in each dish

- Add ½ cup (250ml) of the red kidney beans to each dish

- Add ½ cup (250ml) of the cherry tomatoes to each dish

- Add ½ cup (250ml) of the diced butternut to each dish

- Top each dish with mashed sweet potato, enough to give a generous layer

- Sprinkle 1 tablespoon (15ml) of the seed mix over the top of each dish

- Bake in the oven for 45 minutes

- Since each meal is already in its own serving dish, it can be served straight from the oven.

<u>Snacks</u>

Healthy, well balanced snacks are a very important part of weight and stable blood sugar management. The recipes in this section will give you all the inspiration you need to always have nutritious options to stave off those in-between meal hunger pangs.

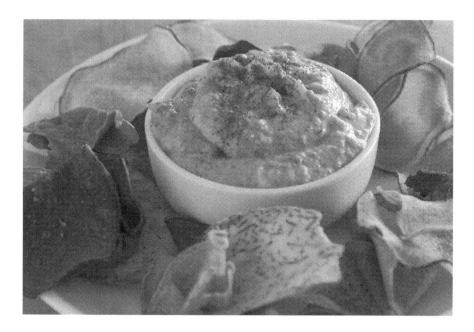

Hummus

Hummus is a great snack option because it is high ... and healthy fats, not to mention that it is incredibly versatile and can be used as an addition to almost any meal. To follow we begin with a basic hummus recipe and then you will find three different variations that will be guaranteed to avoid snack monotony. Each of these recipes makes enough hummus to fill a small medium sized jam jar. These hummus variations are also suitable for home freezing so you could easily freeze smaller portions that will be easy to pre-pack for lunch and snack boxes. When adding hummus as a snack option on its own, its best served with fresh crudités vegetables such as carrot, celery and cucumber sticks. It also goes very well on gluten-free crackers.

Basic Hummus

Ingredients:

- 1 Can Chickpeas, drained and well rinsed

- ¼ Cup (60ml) Tahini

- ¼ Cup (60ml) Freshly squeezed lemon juice

- 1 Teaspoon (5ml) Ground Black Pepper

- 1 Teaspoon (5ml) Organic Ground Sea Salt

- 1 Tablespoon (15ml) Fresh Garlic, finely chopped

Instructions;

1. Using a food processer, place all the ingredients into the bowl

2. Blitz until very smooth

3. You can either store the entire amount in a medium sized glass jar or in smaller containers. However it must be stored in the refrigerator or frozen on the day that you make it.

Basil and Mustard Micro Green Hu

Ingredients:

- 1 Can Chickpeas, drained and well rinsed

- ¼ Cup (60ml) Tahini

- ¼ Cup (60ml) Freshly squeezed lemon juice

- 1 Teaspoon (5ml) Ground Black Pepper

- 1 Teaspoon (5ml) Organic Ground Sea Salt

- 1 Tablespoon (15ml) Fresh Garlic, finely chopped

- 1 Tablespoon (15ml) Fresh Basil, finely chopped

- 1 Tablespoon (15ml) Mustard Micro Greens

Instructions:

1. Using a food processer, place all the ingredients into the bowl

2. Blitz until very smooth

3. You can either store the entire amount in a medium sized glass jar or in smaller containers. However it must be stored in the refrigerator or frozen on the day that you make it.

Curried Hummus

Ingredients:

- 1 Can Chickpeas, drained and well rinsed

- ¼ Cup (60ml) Tahini

- ¼ Cup (60ml) Freshly squeezed lemon juice

- 1 Teaspoon (5ml) Ground Black Pepper

- 1 Teaspoon (5ml) Organic Ground Sea Salt

- 1 Tablespoon (15ml) Fresh Garlic, finely chopped

- 1 Teaspoon (5ml) Gluten-Free Masala mix

- ¼ Teaspoon (1.25ml) Cumin Seeds

Instructions:

1. Using a food processer, place all the ingredients into the bowl

2. Blitz until very smooth

3. You can either store the entire amount in a medium sized glass jar or in smaller containers. However it must be stored in the refrigerator or frozen on the day that you make it.

Coriander and Lime Hummus

Ingredients:

- 1 Can Chickpeas, drained and well rinsed

- ¼ Cup (60ml) Tahini

- ¼ Cup (60ml) Freshly squeezed lime juice

- 1 Teaspoon (5ml) Ground Black Pepper

- 1 Teaspoon (5ml) Organic Ground Sea Salt

- 1 Tablespoon (15ml) Fresh Garlic, finely chopped

- 1 Tablespoon (15ml) Fresh Coriander, finely chopped

- 1 Tablespoon (15ml) Raw Cashew nuts

Instructions:

1. Using a food processer, place all the ingredients into the bowl

2. Blitz until very smooth

3. You can either store the entire amount in a medium sized glass jar or in smaller containers. However it must be stored in the refrigerator or frozen on the day that you make it.

Toasted Chickpeas

a great source of protein, healthy carbohydrates and fiber. This recipe provides you with a much more nutritious option to a bag of commercially made potato chips, that we so often find ourselves grabbing when hunger strikes during a trip to the grocery store. These toasted chickpeas can be made in advance and easily stored in a glass jar or handbag/briefcase sized container. Their tasty crunch is bound to satisfy any snack craving. They also make a great crunchy protein-packed addition to your lunchtime salad.

Makes four ¼ Cup (60ml) servings

Ingredients:

- 1 Can Chickpeas, drained and rinsed

- 1 Teaspoon (5ml) Ground Organic Sea Salt

- 1 Teaspoon (5ml) Ground Black Pepper

- 1 Teaspoon (5ml) Organic dried herb mix

- 1Tablespoon (15ml) Extra Virgin Olive oil

Instructions:

1. Drain and rinse the chickpeas in a colander

2. Pour the chickpeas into a mixing bowl and add the sea salt, black pepper and dried herb mix

3. Toss together well

4. Pour the olive oil over a piece of kitchen paper towel and rub it over a non-stick baking sheet

5. Place the chickpeas onto the baking sheet

6. Turn your oven onto to grill

7. Once the grill element is nice and hot, place the baking sheet with the chickpeas on it under the grill

8. Grill for approximately 25-30minutes, the idea is that the chickpeas lose all their moisture and become browned and crunchy.

Baked Falafel Balls

These falafel balls are another protein-packed, tasty snack option that can be served with any of the above hummus variations. They also make a great protein addition to your lunchtime salad. Because these falafel balls are baked as opposed to the usual method of frying, they are a healthier alternative. Make them in advance and store them in the refrigerator, they can also be frozen.

Makes approximately 45 balls

Ingredients:

- 4 Cans Chickpeas, drained and rinsed

- 2 Teaspoons (10ml) Ground Organic Sea Salt

- 2 Teaspoons (10ml) Ground Black Pepper

- 2 Teaspoons (10ml) Baking Powder

- 1 Teaspoon (5ml) Cumin Seeds

- 1 Teaspoon (5ml) Fresh Coriander, finely chopped

- 1 Teaspoon (5ml) Cayenne Pepper

- 1 Tablespoon (15ml) Fresh Garlic, finely chopped

- 1Tablespoon (15ml) Fresh Ginger root, finely chopped

- ¼ Cup (60ml) Lemon Juice

- ¼ Cup (60ml) Tahini

- 1 Tablespoon (15ml) Extra Virgin Coconut Oil

Instructions:

1. Preheat the oven to 350 degrees (200 degrees Celsius)

2. Place all the ingredients into the food processor and blitz until smooth

3. Place the ingredients into a bowl and refrigerate for about ½ hour, until the mixture has firmed up

4. Using a piece of kitchen paper towel, pour the coconut oil over the paper towel and grease a non-stick baking sheet with it

5. Form the falafel mixture into balls, about the size of a large marble and place the balls onto the baking sheet

6. Bake for 30-35 minutes or until golden brown. Ensure that you turn the balls over half way through cooking.

Fresh Fruit Skewers with Vegan Coconut Yoghurt Dip

Fruit is an incredibly healthy and nutritious snack alternative to sugar laden sweets. The natural sugars in fruits are slowly released and therefore help in maintaining blood sugar without giving you that horrible spike that comes from refined sugar. These skewers are easy to prepare in advance and make a great addition to any lunch box or picnic basket. The coconut yoghurt dip not only adds protein, but also a little extra comfort to this snack combination.

Makes approximately 10 Skewers

Ingredients to make the fruit skewers:

- 1 medium sized fresh papaya, peeled, pitted and cubed

- 1 medium sized fresh pineapple, peeled and cubed

- 1 Cup (250ml) fresh white seedless grapes, whole

- 1 Cup (250ml) fresh black seedless grapes, whole

- 1 Cup (250ml) whole dates

Instructions to make the fruit skewers:

1. Using either wooden or bamboo skewer sticks place the fruit pieces on the skewer sticks, alternating with a

single piece of the different fruits at a time. For example, 1 piece papaya, 1 piece pineapple, 1 white grape, 1 date, 1 red grape.

2. Continue until the skewer is full and then begin the next one

3. Once all the fruit is has been skewered, place the fruit skewers on a serving plate or into a tub for refrigeration.

Ingredients to make the vegan yoghurt dip:

- 1 Cup (250ml) vegan coconut yogurt (or other vegan yoghurt of your choice)

- ¼ Cup (60ml) Coconut Cream

- 1 Teaspoon (5ml) Vanilla Essence

- ½ Teaspoon (2.5ml) Ground Cinnamon

- 1 Teaspoon (5ml) Raw Cocoa Powder

- 1 Tablespoon (15ml) Desiccated Coconut

- 1 Tablespoon (15ml) Dried Berry mix

Instructions to make the yoghurt dip:

1. Place the yoghurt and coconut cream into a mixing bowl

2. Add the vanilla essence, ground cinnamon and raw cocoa powder

3. Whisk well

4. Stir in the desiccated coconut and the dried berry mix

5. If you are serving the fruit skewers at home then place the yoghurt dip into a serving dish. If you are taking the skewers to go, then place the yoghurt dip into a take away container. Both the yoghurt dip and the fruit skewers are best kept refrigerated, so if you are taking them in your lunch box or to a picnic, ensure that they are in a cooler bag.

Homemade Trail Mix

Trail mix is another great on-the-go snack option, often the pre-packed versions that we buy in the supermarkets contain unnecessary additives and preservatives. By mixing your own trail mix, using organic, raw ingredients you are ensuring that you get a healthy, energy-boosting snack that you can trust. This recipe includes dried berry mix and raw cocoa nibs, making it a great source of anti-oxidants as well.

Makes approximately 4 ¼ Cup (60ml) Servings

Ingredients:

- 4 Tablespoons (60ml) Raw Cashew Nuts, whole

- 4 Tablespoons (60ml) Raw Brazil Nuts, Whole

- 4 Tablespoons (60ml) Raw Seed mix

- 4 Tablespoons (60ml) Dried Berry Mix

- 4 Tablespoons (60ml) Coconut Flakes

- 4 Tablespoons (60ml) Raw Cocoa Nibs

- 4 Tablespoons (60ml) Dried Mango Pieces

- 4 Tablespoons (60ml) Dried Apple Pieces

structions:

1. Place all the ingredients into a large mixing bowl and toss together well

2. Using a ¼ cup (60ml) measuring cup, divide the trail mix into portions

3. You can either place each portion in a small sandwich bag, or a small take away tub.

4. If you choose not to pre-portion out the entire mix, then you can store it in an airtight glass jar.

Your Free Gift

Don't forget to download your free complimentary recipe eBook:

Click here or visit:

http://bit.ly/VeganSmoothiesKaren

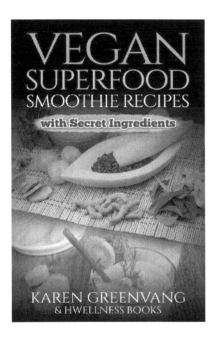

If you have any problems with your download, email me at: karenveganbooks@gmail.com

Conclusion

Thank you for reading!

I hope that with so many vegan-gluten free friendly recipes you will be motivated and inspired to start your journey towards meaningful veganism, vibrant health and total wellbeing.

Remember, the beauty of incorporating nutritious vegan foods into your daily diet is that you are making simple, yet sustainable changes that will work for your wellness long-term. Not to mention your spiritual wellness and taking care of the environment.

If you enjoyed my book, it would be greatly appreciated if you left a review so others can receive the same benefits you have. Your review can help other people take this important step to take care of their health and inspire them to start a new chapter in their lives.

At the same time, you can help me serve you and all my other readers even more through my next vegan-friendly recipe books that I am committed to publishing on a regular basis.

I'd be thrilled to hear from you. I would love to know your favorite recipe(s).

Don't be shy, post a comment on Amazon!

→ Questions about this book? Email me at: karenveganbooks@gmail.com

Thank You for your time,

Love & Light,

Until next time-

Karen Vegan Greenvang

More Vegan Books by Karen

Available in kindle and paperback in all Amazon stores

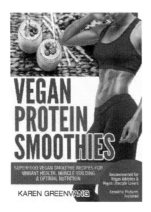

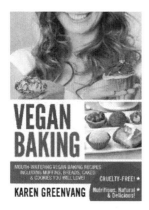

You will find more at:

www.amazon.com/author/karengreenvang

Made in the USA
Middletown, DE
24 August 2018